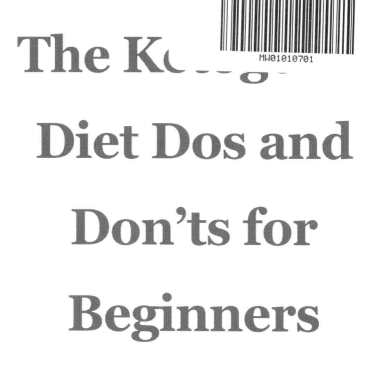

The Ketogenic Diet Dos and Don'ts for Beginners

How to Lose Weight and Feel Amazing

Mathew Noll

© 2016

TABLE OF CONTENTS

INTRODUCTION

The Ketogenic diet is not a new concept in the world of losing weight. However, to follow this path is definitely something which requires due consideration time and again. You cannot just lose weight by abiding a list of foods that are prescribed in any diet plan. You need to take care of many other things despite taking all other precautions.

THE KETOGENIC DIET DOS AND DON'TS FOR BEGINNERS: How to Lose Weight and Feel Amazing has been written so as to focus only and only on weight loss. You will not find any other information that is not relevant to the topic. There are many people who have benefitted from the Ketogenic diet. However, there are some others too who have been following this amazing diet plan by heart, but are still not able to lose weight. If you belong to the latter category, this book is for you.

There are many things in your body which do not let you lose weight, including your habits. You need to work on everything simultaneously for a long time, not necessary for everyone though, to lose those extra inches on your body. Persistently working on one regime definitely gives you the results you want.

You might have come across real life examples of people, who used to live for carbohydrates. But, when they quit those foods, they did it forever. That is what is asked for in a real life change and your body fat vanishes permanently. Get inspired from such people and start your own regime of the Ketogenic diet. Go ahead with this book and we wish you all the luck to have a body that you always wanted.

CHAPTER 1

What is the Ketogenic Diet?

You might have heard your friends talking about ketosis, the Ketogenic diet, etc. And, here you are researching about what they are talking about so passionately. The Ketogenic diet has now become well known for losing weight through a strange phenomenon. It is called strange because for some people depending upon fats for losing fats sounds astonishing! We cannot normally imagine that we have to eat the same thing that we want to eliminate from our body - fats!

The Ketogenic diet consists of high amounts of fats, ample proteins and fewer carbohydrates. It forces the body to use fats instead of carbs for breaking down to convert them into energy. In our regular diets, we consume more carbohydrate and shun fats. Thus, our body is perfectly adapted throughout history to break down carbohydrates for energy. However, in the Ketogenic diet, we try to change the pattern of our body to break down the elements to be used for energy. We feed our body with more fats and less carbohydrates and thus force it to adapt in a new way to use fats for energy.

The plus side to this diet is that you do not have to count your calories or the amount of fats you are consuming like the way you do in other diets. You can indulge in different types of meats and oils, do not feel guilty and still lose weight. You must be wondering how it is possible. In the next few chapters you will discover how.

Normally, our body would convert food into glucose that would be transported to various body parts. This glucose is especially important in fueling functions of the brain. It is easiest for your body to convert carbs into glucose and use it as energy. Thus, it is obvious that your body will choose carbs over any other source of energy. Our body produces insulin to process glucose in the bloodstream and makes it travel around the body. Since glucose is there to provide energy to your body, fats are not required and hence, stored.

However, if you do not feed your body with carbohydrates, the liver starts converting fats to ketone bodies and fatty acids. These ketone bodies enter the brain and pass through it to replace the old source of energy, which was glucose. Thus, all the fats you consume in the form of meats, oils, creams, etc. is broken down and it does not get accumulated in your body. When you lower down the carbs intake, the body is persuaded to enter into a state of ketosis. It is just a natural process, which is initiated by the body to help it survive when the food consumption is low.

The Ketogenic diet is known by some other names as well- low carbs high fat diet (LCHF), low carb diet. The ultimate aim of a well maintained Ketogenic diet is to persuade the body into a metabolic state. But, this does not mean that you have to go hungry on calories. However, you just have to strictly control your consumption of carbohydrates. It is definitely easier than starving on fats.

Human body is extremely adaptive to everything it is forced into. If you make it depend on a new source of energy rather than the regular one, it will adapt accordingly in a few days.

CHAPTER 2

Before You Start the Ketogenic Diet

If you have been looking for something simple that can be followed to lose weight, you are reading the right thing. Just one month into the Ketogenic diet will give you best results that you would have never seen in any other diet.

You may read or hear sometimes that you do not have to count calories in the Ketogenic diet. However, it is better that you do. Mostly, the high intake of fats and just adequate intake of proteins would be sufficient to keep you naturally satiated and also keep you away from carbohydrates. However, in America, this is not so simple. You have to consider enormous amount of endocrine, hormones and problems of deficiency. Your body would not be able to lose weight if you feed it more than it consumes.

Have you heard of "macros"? It is an abbreviated name for macronutrients, which are carbs, proteins and fats. You need to find out first what amount of macros does your body need to achieve your goals. You can use some online calculators to find out the same if you know a few intricate details about macros. Else, you can also take the help of your physician to determine the level of proteins, carbs and fats that your body needs.

Many people consider the level of macros as if they have been written in stone. You do not have to worry about achieving the set marks every day. It is totally fine that you overachieve or underachieve your targets. In the long term, everything is going to be fine. The Ketogenic diet is a plan for long term, not the opposite of it.

An average woman would require 74 grams of proteins, 136 grams of fats and 20 grams of carbohydrates per day in the Ketogenic diet. This requirement of an average female body is based on a sedentary lifestyle. Now, if you want to decrease or increase the amount of calories, you can do it if your body demands so.

It is quite easy to increase calories - you just need to increase the quantity of fats you consume. Consuming coconut oil, olive oil, butter and macadamia nuts is a healthy and simple way to increase the amount of fats that you take. You can sprinkle these oils on salads, snack on them, mix them with vegetables or consume them however you like.

However, if you want to decrease the calories, you would have to reflect upon it a lot and think of alternatives so that your body does not fall short of energy. Most probably, you will have to cut down on proteins also. Thus, you need to keep in mind the sized portions of your meals. Increase them or decrease them as you see fit.

The most important thing in the end is the stick to the Ketogenic diet. The process of ketosis constantly happens in your body. When your body starts depending on fats for energy, you cannot just "cheat once" on your meals. If you still do, it implies that you would ruin your efforts that you did in the past one week with just one cheat meal! It will take another one week to take your body back to ketosis and function normally again.

You would definitely never want to cheat if you are fully determined. You have to be mentally prepared and gear up your kitchen with all the groceries of the Ketogenic diet. Be prepared with what you want to eat and what you need to eat. The food you eat must keep you satiated as well as mentally satisfied. If you forcefully eat something, you are bound to cheat or fail in the long term. When you go through the diet charts of the Ketogenic diet, decide for yourself what you like to eat and do not hesitate to try new meats and other foods. You never know, you might fall in love with them.

CHAPTER 3

How to Lose Weight with the Ketogenic Diet?

Are you facing trouble shedding weight? Or are you not satisfied by the pace you are losing weight? Do not worry. Now that you have chosen the Ketogenic diet for your weight loss program, you have taken the perfect step.

You would have heard it a zillion times that you need to eat less and work out more to lose weight. However, these ideas are not sustainable in the long term. You might have been counting your calories, working out for hours each day and trying to suppress your hunger. Now is the time that you mark a full stop to those endless times of suffering. Such efforts waste your willpower and your time as well. Most diet plans make you suffer. That is why you notice so many people around you who are obese and their current position of the body is the result of continuous failed diets.

Fortunately, we have a better option. The Ketogenic diet works in such a manner that you do not have to make much conscious efforts. The Ketogenic diet hormonally regulates your weight. The only thing necessary to lose weight is to reduce the amount of insulin in your body, which works to store fat. When you successfully cut down the amount of insulin, you do not have to make excess efforts to lose weight.

Read further to know how you can shed off that extra fat on your waist and thighs.

1. Choose a diet containing fewer carbohydrates

You need to cut down on your consumption of starch and sugar. This idea is more than a century old. There have been a lot of diet plans which are based on reducing the amount of carbs you take. The new thing with the Ketogenic diet is that you provide your body with an alternate source of energy to depend on, which is fats.

The science behind any weight loss regime is that you should consume lesser calories than your body can burn. The only issue with this basic advice is that you ignore the elephant in the room- your hunger. Almost all of us would agree on this fact that you cannot just eat less food and stay hungry forever. You are not a masochist, right? When you starve too much, you tend to "cheat" again and again. The Ketogenic diet makes you "want" to consume less food. There are many overweight people who do not even count their calories and still eat fewer calories because they do not *want* to eat them. Starch and sugar may raise your hunger levels and if you avoid it, you may decrease your desire for food to an inadequate level. Your body might require more calories than you are feeding it with. In that case, you do not need to specifically count them.

When you do not eat carbohydrates or eat them moderately, your body is capable of burning 300 additional calories per day, even when you are resting! It means that this amount of burnt calories is equal to a gym session of moderate physical activity.

The bottom line is that the Ketogenic diet reduces your need for food naturally and you do not have to hog food all day. Thus, you naturally eat less without starving. Moreover, your body keeps burning fats even when you are not exercising.

2. Eat when you feel hungry

You do not need to stay hungry all the time to lose weight. This is the most common mistake committed by people who start a low carb diet. In the Ketogenic diet, you do not have to be scared of fats. Carbohydrates and fats are two major sources of energy for our body. If you are snatching carbs from your body, you need to give it an ample supply of fats. Low fats and low carbs equal to starvation, and we do not want that, do we? Starvation results in cravings and fatigue. That is why, people who starve give up easily on their diet plans. The better solution is to consume natural fat till the time you are satisfied. Some of the natural fats are full fat cream, butter, olive oil, meat, bacon, fatty fish, coconut oil, eggs.

You must always eat enough in order to feel satisfied, particularly when you start your regime of weight loss. When you eat enough fats, your body would not look for carbs to use them for energy. In other words, when your body does not have insulin that stores fat, you become a fat burning engine. You will start losing weight without feeling hungry.

Are you scared of saturated fat? You don't have to. The obsolete theories which stated that saturated fat is not good for health have been disapproved by modern science. Saturated fats are fine foods.

Eating when you are hungry implies that you do not have to push food down your throat if you are not hungry. You need to trust your instincts of satiety and hunger. Also, if you feel hungry several times a day, feel free to indulge in your favorite saturated fats meals.

Some people would eat thrice a day and take snacks between the meals too. There is another set of people who would just eat twice a day and do not snack at all. Do not go by the eating patterns of others. Follow whatever suits your body. Just remember one thumb rule that you must eat whenever you feel hungry.

3. Eat real food

This is one more common mistake made by Ketogenic followers that they get fooled by the fraudulent but creative marketing of "low-carb" foods. A real Ketogenic diet should be supported by real food. It implies the food which is being eaten by humans for millions of years. For example, fish, meat, vegetables, olive oil, butter, nuts, etc.

If you are truly determined to lose weight, you must avoid falling in the trap of those products which claim to be low on carbs, but are actually high on carbs. It is obvious that the food industry has been fooling around with people on diet to transfer money from the consumer's pocket to their own. You would hear many brands claiming that you can eat pasta, cookies, bread, and as much chocolate as you want with their brand. Do not get fooled because these products are full of carbohydrates!

What do you think about the low-carbs bread? Do you really think that it is low on carbs? It is not, despite all the claims made by the companies. Anything made of grains, plus baked is certainly not a low carbs food.

You must have heard of low-carbs chocolate. They usually contain sugar alcohol, the element which is not counted by the manufacturers are carbohydrates but is certainly not good for your process of ketosis. The excess amount of carbs from such processed foods result in colon, which causes diarrhea and gas.

In brief, just follow these two thumb rules:

- Do not consume "low carbs" adaptation of these high carbs foods like bars, cookies, bread, pasta, ice cream, etc. You can rather make these things yourself to be sure of ingredients.

- You must avoid food that says "net carbs" in description. This is just another way to trap you. Avoid processed foods.

Also, you must buy stuff that does not have a long list of ingredients. This list must be very short, if you essentially have to buy processed foods.

4. Eat *only* if you feel hungry

You must have read tip number 2 above. In the Ketogenic diet, eat when you are hungry. Do not eat when you are not feeling hungry. Let us elaborate why we are stressing this point again. Unnecessary snacking may become a mammoth issue in the Ketogenic diet. Some products are just so easily available and they are so tempting that you cannot resist them. Watch out for these three traps:

- **Dairy products:** Eating cheese is not prohibited in the Ketogenic diet. But, if you eat too much of it while watching TV, even when you are not hungry; it will not let you lose weight at all. If you are already full, resist putting too much cream on your dessert. Avoid putting too much cream in your coffee several times a day.

- **Nuts:** You might have gobbled down the nuts in the bowl until all of them are gone, no matter your stomach is already full. If you eat unsalted nuts, you can resist overeating them. Thus, now you know one wiser thing to do. Buy unsalted, raw nuts. Also, do not take the whole packet of nuts to your couch. Put them in a small bowl and sit down to eat.

- **LCHF baking:** Yes, we know that you are going to use natural sweeteners and almond flour in your cookies and sweet bombs. But, overindulging in these snacks is also not a wise thing to do.

You can skip meals

Yes, you heard it right. You can even skip breakfast if you are not feeling hungry. This holds truth for any meal. When you are strictly following the Ketogenic diet, your hunger goes down significantly, especially if you have to lose a lot of weight. Your body is happily busy in burning excess fats and reduces your temptation to eat.

Thus, do not get scared that you will get weak if you do not eat! Your body has sufficient fats to burn for energy even if you do not eat. You must wait for feeling happily hungry. You will save both money and time and speed up your process of weight loss. You do not have to be obsessed with food and snack every hour. Remember that you are not on a high carbs diet.

5. Wisely measure your development

Losing weight successfully might get trickier sometimes. If you focus on your weight all the time and step on the weighing scale all the time, you may get mislead. It de-motivates you and makes you anxious needlessly.

The weighing scale does not give the exact measure of the shape of your body. It measures your internal organs, bones and muscles also. Gaining muscles is good for your body. BMI or body mass index is a more appropriate method to track your progress.

If you have begun weight training or you have been gaining muscles, your fat loss may get hidden. Do not get mislead if you do not notice any major changes in your body weight. You can rather measure the circumference of your waist and cheer up over the loss of belly fat. You can have a decent belly if you are a middle aged person with the Ketogenic diet. It is easier for younger people to lose belly fat.

Measure progress

You can measure the circumference of your waist and your

weight before you start the Ketogenic diet and then do it weekly or even monthly. Do not do it too often. Maintain a journal to write these results. You can also measure your hips, chest, legs and arms.

It is important to remember that your weight may swing up and down, depending upon the balance of fluids and the contents of stomach. Do not get anxious over short term fluctuations. Ponder over the results of long term.

You must also keep a track of the following elements too:

- Blood sugar
- Blood pressure
- Profile of cholesterol

The Ketogenic diet approves low carbs foods and these markers make sure that you remain in good health while losing weight. You should keep checking these markers after a few months. It is important to gain health also while losing weight.

6. Be persistent
You would have all those chunks of fats around your waist and

thighs in several years. So, how do you expect to lose all the extra fat in just a few weeks? If you want to shed that extra weight permanently, you have to make persistent efforts.

What you should aim for?

You would definitely lose 4-6 pounds in the first week of your Ketogenic diet. Then, about 1 pound is lost every week on an average. You can say it like you might lose 50 pounds every year. 5 pounds lost mean that your waist would lose 1 inch in circumference. Young men lose weight much faster than average. However, women after menopause may lose weight slightly slowly.

You can exercise vigorously if you do not have the patience to wait for a year or so. As you come closer to the ideal body weight, the process of weight loss slows down until your weight stabilizes. You will never go underweight with the Ketogenic diet till the time you consume fats whenever you feel hungry. You do not need to starve under any circumstances.

Stalls in the beginning

You may not notice your body losing weight in the initial phase of this diet. But, do not lose focus and be persistent.

Plateaus of weight loss

There might be some weeks or days at a stretch when you do not notice any changes in your body. Keep calm and do not leave your routine. The changes will occur sooner or later.

Lose excess weight permanently

You have to change your habits permanently to lose excess weight eternally. If you achieve your ideal state of a perfect body you always wanted, but return to your old habits, you are doomed to gain weight again. Do not be shocked at that time. It requires a lot of patience to have a perfect body. There are no quick fixes for quick weight loss. They are all scams if you have ever heard of any such quick fixes.

Moreover, only the initial phase of a long term change is difficult. It's like quitting an addiction of drugs. Once you build up new habits, you will find it easier every passing day to stick to your healthy routine. It happens naturally.

7. Women should avoid savoring fruits

For women, fruit is more of an obstacle to lose weight. Yes, it is true. The same is true for men as well, but for women on

Ketogenic diet, fruits may prove a major impediment in their already demanding journey. You may find it controversial when we say that you should not eat fruits, especially when the status of fruits has achieved a magical aura for health today.

You already know that most fruits contain 90% of water. The remaining weight of fruits is sugar and only sugar. You can recall many fruits like grapes, pears, oranges - they are all sweet, aren't they? If you take five portions of fruits everyday; they are equal to the quantity of sugar contained in 500 ml of soda (16 ounces). And this sugar is more or less similar to artificial sugar we consume (50% fructose, 50% glucose).

Thus, now you may understand that the sugar contained in the fruits may stop the process of burning of fats in your body. It may increase your hunger and thus, slow down your burning of calories. You can enjoy your favorite fruits occasionally as a treat but do not eat them daily.

8. Men must avoid beer

Like fruits, beer is also an impediment in losing weight. It is equally true for women too, but it has been specifically said for men because men drink more beer frequently. Beer consists of rapidly digested carbohydrates which shut down burning of fats. You might have heard of beer being called 'liquid bread" in some of the parties. Fat people are even referred to have a "beer belly"!

You can drink some other kinds of alcohol if you want to get high and still lose weight:

- Red wine or dry white wine
- Dry champagne
- Vodka, cognac, whiskey and other pure spirits

You must keep away from sweetened cocktails. You can rather take vodka, lime and soda instead. Hard drinks mentioned above have extremely low content of sugar and carbohydrates. Thus, they are a definitely better option than beer. But, this does not mean that you can drink these drinks like a fish and still remain self complacent that you are going well. If you drink too much of alcohol, your weight loss process is definitely going to slow down. Thus, drinking in moderation can be fine.

9. Stay away from artificial sugars

If you have been relying the luring ads of artificial sweeteners and have gave them the space of sugar in your kitchen, you are doing nothing but fooling yourself. You might think that artificial sweeteners reduce your calorie intake. However, this is an absolute myth and these products do not help to lose weight.

There had been many studies being done to find out the authenticity of claims made by the advertisements of artificial sweeteners. But, they failed to find any evidence which proved that consuming these products in place of plain sugar have any effect on burning fats

In fact, there have been some studies, which suggest that artificial sweeteners are capable of increasing your appetite. They even keep up your carving for other sweet products. You can put purified water in your drinks instead, which naturally is a little sweet in taste, to lose weight.

The reason behind the worthiness of artificial sweeteners may be that our body secretes more insulin when we drink something that contains artificial sweetener. But, since no sugar enters our body to meet with insulin, the level of blood sugar drops and we suddenly feel hungrier. However, it happens every time or not, it is not yet clear.

Harmful effects of artificial sweeteners

Artificial sweeteners are the proven culprits of maintaining the sweet product addiction and also result in craving of snacks. However, there are no concrete studies on the long term side effects of these products since they have not been in the market for too long.

The studies that claim positive or neutral effects of artificial sweeteners are normally sponsored by the beverage industry. If you have decided to positively lose weight, you must avoid every kind of sweeteners. The plus side of this practice is that you will fall in love with the natural sweet flavor of real foods.

10. Check your medications

There are many prescription drugs that can stall your process of weight loss. You must tell your doctor that you are on a weight loss regime and thus, he must not prescribe any such drugs which may make you gain weight. Here are some of the medications which you must consume carefully:

Insulin Injections: When they are taken in higher dose, they can become the very bad impediment for losing weight. You can reduce your requirement for insulin by eating lesser carbohydrates. After the discussion with your doctor, you can take 2-3 grams per day of Metmorfin tablets for type 2 diabetes. This type of diabetes is also curable with Byetta or Victoza in place of insulin. However, the long term effects of these medicines are not yet known.

There are some **anti-depressant medicines** which can lead to weight gain. Also, some **contraceptives** are also the culprit for the same. Medicines for **blood pressure, epilepsy drugs, allergy medicines, antibiotics** are also some of the major contributors for weight gain.

11. Take Less Stress and More Sleep

You might have thought many times that if you could have less stress in life and some more hours of sleep, your life would be better. Well, if this happens with you regularly, this is not good news for weight loss. However, it is never too late. The Ketogenic diet cannot work alone with eating this and not eating that. You have to take care of other factors as well.

Chronic stress increases the levels of Cortisol, which is a stress hormone, in your body. It may increase your hunger levels and thus, you may gain weight rather than lose it. You must find out ways to decrease stress and have a peaceful deep sleep daily. Also, try to wake up fresh without depending on your alarm clock. An alarm clock wakes you up brutally and thus, stresses you early in the morning.

A very efficient method to fight this struggle is to sleep early and wake up on your own before the alarm bell rings. This will not only reduce stress in your mind, but also allow you to wake up fresh.

Another aspect of taking less sleep is that it also affects your self-discipline adversely. When you want to stop yourself from eating sugar, the stress on your mind will not let you do so. It also does not let you wake up for work out. You must stick to a fixed time of sleeping. Avoid taking coffee or caffeine in any other form after 2 pm. Also, do not take alcohol 3 hours prior to sleeping. Alcohol interferes with your quality of sleep. That is why; you wake up tired after a night of boozing. If you have to work out in the evening, do it at least 4 hours before sleeping. Also, ensure that your bedroom is maintained at a pleasant temperature and there is sufficient darkness at the time of sleeping.

12. Attain optimal ketosis

If, even after taking all the precautions and eating in line with the diet chart of the Ketogenic diet, you are not able to lose weight as you want you need to attain the state of optimal ketosis. Sometimes, you might reach a weight plateau, where your weight just stabilizes and does not go down further. At such times, optimal ketosis can be helpful.

In the Ketogenic diet, your body is modified to eat less carbs, adequate proteins and more fat. But, how do you know that this diet is efficiently working for your body? The answer is - optimal ketosis.

What is ketosis?

Ketosis refers to that state when your body burns fat at extremely high rate. Even your brain starts functioning with the help of ketone bodies. To encourage the production of ketone, insulin levels in your body should be low. When the ketone bodies are sufficiently higher to help to lose weight quickly, the state is called optimal ketosis.

How to measure ketone bodies?

You can easily find gadgets in the market that are specially meant for measuring ketone bodies. And, they are not very expensive. You just need to prick your finger with a needle and you can determine the ketone level in your blood instantly. This test should be done on a fasting stomach early in the morning. You can take the help of the following chart to check your results:

- If the result shows below 0.5 millimoles per liter, you are too far from ketosis.
- If it is between 0.5-1.5 millimoles per liter, you have achieved light nutritional ketosis. You still need to work on your weight loss despite losing a few pounds.
- If the results show it approximately 1.5-3 millimoles per liter, this state is known as optimal ketosis. At this stage, you can lose maximum weight.

The results over 3 millimoles per liter are not required. They will not have any effects more than optimal ketosis. In fact, if the values come out too high, it means that you are not taking sufficient food.

Urine test

The level of ketone can also be measured by a urine test. The urine test sticks come cheap and are readily available at the pharmacies. However, their results are not very accurate for different reasons.

How to attain optimal ketosis?

Just eating very low quantities of carbohydrates is not enough to achieve optimal ketosis. Do not get upset. You just need to control your diet of proteins as well. If you consume too many eggs, meat or anything that contains high amounts of proteins, the ketone levels may not reach the appropriate level. The excess amount of protein gets changed into glucose. Insulin level may also get high with proteins. All these factors compromise on achieving optimal ketosis.

The key to avoid all these obstacles is to consume as much fat as possible to avoid pangs of hunger. If you eat a heavy breakfast full of fats, you will not feel hungry at least till lunch. This will make sure that you stick to your diet and do not munch on carbs or proteins. That will be when your weight plateau will be replaced by optimal ketosis.

Beware

If you are a patient of type 1 diabetes, it is not at all suggested that you follow the advices mentioned above. It might prove extremely risky for your health. You need to consult your doctor before you proceed with the Ketogenic diet plans.

13. Get yourself tested for your hormones makeup

Even after following all the above tips, you are not able to reach the desired state of weight; you must consider hormonal imbalance in your body. The most common areas of problems are:

- Sex hormones
- Thyroid hormones
- Stress hormones

Sex Hormones

They are also responsible in regulating your weight. Insulin and testosterone levels are often imbalanced in women due to endocrine disorder. The common results are weight gain, menstrual disorders, acne, infertility and hair growth like men, especially on the face. The LCFH diet like the Ketogenic diet is a good cure for these problems.

After middle age, the male sex hormone, testosterone, and the female sex hormone, estrogen, declines. This leads to weight gain and a decrease in muscle mass. You can keep up your sex hormones by indulging in exercise routines, checking your body language and a good intake of Vitamin D. However, you should check with your doctor that your levels of sex hormones are not too high for your age. Otherwise, it may result in breast cancer in women and prostate cancer in men.

Thyroid Hormone

An imbalance of thyroid hormones decreases the rate of metabolism. The result is a condition called hypothyroidism, which shows symptoms like cold intolerance, fatigue, constipation, weight gain, dry skin. Normally, the weight gain in such conditions is up to 15 pounds. Get yourself tested for thyroid hormones. To avoid their deficiency, you can do the following:

- Ensure that you consume enough iodine. Iodine can be consumed from sources like shellfish, fish and sea salt or iodized salt.
- With the advice of your doctor, you can take supplements of a thyroid hormone.

"Hypothyroidism Type 2"

You might get diagnosed with "Hypothyroidism Type 2" if you have been experiencing fatigue or other symptoms despite your thyroid hormone levels are normal. A healthcare expert might even recommend supplements. You need to be skeptical at this time. It might mask several other health issues in your body. Overdose of a thyroid hormone may imbalance other hormones in your body. It is obvious that you might feel energetic with the supplements in the short term, but they are definitely not healthy in the long term.

Stress hormone

Cortisol, the stress hormone, is the ultimate culprit behind the failure of your efforts. We have already discussed how stress may become a hindrance in losing weight. Thus, you must work on reducing stress so that your efforts of losing weight do not go waste.

CONCLUSION

Most of us have excess weight on our body and we want to lose it forever. Some of us can achieve it easily and for the others, it is a mammoth task, which is next to impossible. But, there is one thing you must never forget - Do not lose heart ever! Losing weight is just a small thing in front of many which you need to accomplish in your life. If you are determined to do it, no one can stop you.

In **THE KETOGENIC DIET DOS AND DON'TS FOR BEGINNERS: How to Lose Weight and Feel Amazing,** you would have found many tips that are useful for you and many more which you would have thought that you already knew. The purpose of writing this book was to remind you of some things which you might have forgotten with time and to let you know some other things which are necessary for losing weight.

But, whatever efforts you make to shed those extra pounds which you think are unnecessary, you must take your age into consideration. If you have crossed the middle age, you must wisely accept that you should not and cannot have the body like that of a 16 year old kid. If you have crossed that stage of youthfulness when you enjoyed your body more than anything, now is the time to just shed the extra weight and gain good health. You must both aim for a healthy lifestyle and try to be grateful and happy for the body that you are given.

Sometimes, in the rage of achieving perfection for our body, we forget to be grateful for what we have- a healthy body. Many people don't even have a complete body. Thus, we would really suggest that you do aim for perfection but do not forget to have the much needed gratitude. It keeps you both healthy and happy.

Have a great life!

Made in the USA
San Bernardino, CA
12 January 2019